Medicinal Mushrooms

THE ESSENTIAL GUIDE

by Martin Powell

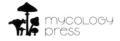

mycology press

First published in 2013 by Mycology Press, an imprint of Bamboo Publishing Ltd.

ISBN 978-0-9566898-1-8

Book Design by CreativeCo Ltd
35A Monument Business Park, Chalgrove, Oxfordshire OX44 7RW

Contents

Preface

For thousands of years mushrooms have been valued by cultures around the world for their therapeutic potential as well as for their nutritional value and *Medicinal Mushrooms – The Essential Guide* is designed as a resource for the layperson wishing to understand more about the health benefits of these remarkable organisms.

In order to make the information as accessible as possible technical detail has been kept to a minimum and those looking for a more detailed treatment of the subject are referred to *Medicinal Mushrooms – A Clinical Guide* (pub. 2010).

Rather than an exhaustive list of every mushroom, or of all the research on each mushroom, I have opted to focus on ten of the most prominent medicinal mushrooms and the main areas in which they can have a real impact on our health.

In the same way, I have not listed every compound found in every mushroom but have chosen to focus on the main classes of compound responsible for the health benefits of each mushroom.

For ease of access references are given with the title first.

Martin Powell
Eastbourne – August 2013

About the Author

Martin Powell is a biochemist and Chinese herbalist who has worked with mushroom nutrition for over 20 years. He lectures at the University of Westminster and is the author of *Medicinal Mushrooms – A Clinical Guide*.

As well as running a clinical practice, he continues to research mushrooms' health benefits and runs seminars on their clinical use for doctors and other healthcare practitioners in the UK and worldwide.

Disclaimer

The information contained in this book is presented for educational use only and is not meant to be used, nor should it be used, to diagnose or treat any medical condition. Anyone who is experiencing any symptoms, has been diagnosed with or suspects they may have a medical condition should contact a medical doctor or other appropriately qualified health professional. The reader should not assume that because an adverse reaction or interaction is not mentioned in this book the use of any given medicinal mushroom is always safe. If you suspect you could be experiencing an adverse reaction from a mushroom or a combination of mushroom(s) and drugs, you should immediately consult an appropriately qualified health professional. Likewise, you should always inform your healthcare provider of any supplements you may be taking. Both the author and publisher accept neither liability nor responsibility to any person with respect to loss, injury or damage caused, or alleged to be caused, directly or indirectly by the information contained in this book.

Introduction

Traditionally valued for their health benefits as well as their nutritional value, modern research is now confirming the therapeutic properties of many mushroom species.

In addition, mushrooms are proving a rich source of physiologically active compounds with extracts from over 650 mushrooms having been shown to have immunological activity, while evidence from epidemiological studies points to a significant correlation between increased mushroom intake and reduced risk of serious illness, including cancer[1,3].

How Medicinal Mushrooms Work

Mushrooms are part of the fungal kingdom. As such they are more closely related to humans and other members of the animal kingdom than to plants and, partly because of this relative evolutionary closeness, many of the compounds they produce show physiological activity in humans as well as other animals.

In some cases these compounds can be harmful, hence the caution required when harvesting mushrooms from the wild, but in many cases they offer significant health benefits. Indeed, many of the top-selling pharmaceutical products are derived from mushrooms and other fungi, including the major antibiotics as well as statin-class compounds, such as Lovastatin and Simvastatin.

Of course mushrooms do not produce these compounds for our benefit but rather to give themselves an advantage in the competition with other micro-organisms for food and resources and as such many show anti-microbial activity, either as antibiotics or as anti-fungal agents[4].

At the same time, as our immune system has evolved, it has done so alongside fungal pathogens and has developed the ability to recognise many of the structural components of the mushroom cell wall as foreign, with at least seven receptors on the surface of major classes of immune cell binding specifically to mushroom cell-wall compounds[5].

Active Compounds from Medicinal Mushrooms

Immunologically active polysaccharides and related compounds	Anti-microbial compounds and other secondary metabolites
Found in all mushrooms	*Differ from species to species*

The majority of these compounds are polysaccharide-based, usually with bound protein components. Although often referred to as beta-glucans (or 1-3,1-6 beta-glucans), in reality they contain a wide range of sugars in diverse configurations[6].

Binding of mushroom polysaccharide to the different immune receptors triggers widespread immunological changes with increases in activity of key categories of immune cells, helping to restore healthy immune function and facilitating an effective immune response to pathogenic fungi, other micro-organisms or cancer cells[7].

Importantly, although the effect of mushroom polysaccharides is to help restore immune competency in individuals whose immune system is compromised by stress, chronic illness or tumour burden, in individuals with auto-immune conditions and whose immune system is overactive, mushroom polysaccharides help to restore balance by down-regulating key components of the pro-inflammatory immune response.

This ability of mushroom polysaccharides to help restore healthy balance to the immune system, up-regulating immune responses in cases of immune suppression while down-regulating overactive immune responses, is a direct consequence of their being natural compounds that our immune system has learned to recognize and respond to appropriately over millions of years and makes them a uniquely suitable food for a wide range of chronic health conditions[8].

Immunological changes triggered by mushroom polysaccharides

- Activation of immune cells such as: macrophages, neutrophils, monocytes, Natural Killer cells (NK cells) and dendritic cells
- Increased antibody production
- Increased interferon production
- Increased immune system activity against a range of cancers
- Inhibition of tumour metastasis
- Reduction in pro-inflammatory cytokines
- Inhibition of prostaglandin synthesis

Using Medicinal Mushrooms

Many of the mushrooms that fall into the medicinal mushroom category are also delicious culinary mushrooms and, as most of the active compounds they contain are not adversely affected by cooking, their health benefits can in many cases be enjoyed by including them as part of a balanced diet, either in fresh or dried form (although needing rehydration, dried mushrooms offer almost the same health benefits as fresh mushrooms).

In cases where higher concentrations of key active components are desired, or where regular dietary consumption is difficult, a growing number of mushroom supplements are also available. These may be based on the mushroom as we eat it, ie. the above-ground fruiting body, or they may be derived from cultivated versions of the fine, thread-like filaments or hyphae (mycelium) found in the substrate from which the fruiting bodies emerge.

Types of Mushroom Supplement

- Fruiting body – Dried and powdered fruiting bodies.
- Mycelium (liquid fermentation) – Grown using the same liquid fermentation technology used to produce penicillin etc. 100% mushroom material. In some cases supplements also contain culture-medium filtrates to capture compounds secreted by the growing mushroom.
- Mycelial Biomass (solid fermentation) – Grown by inoculating a sterile, grain-based substrate with mushroom mycelium. As well as mushroom mycelium, contains residual enzymatically-transformed substrate, together with extra-cellular components, especially anti-microbial compounds, secreted by the mycelium into the substrate. Also referred to as 'full-spectrum'.
- Hot-water extracts – These can be derived from either the fruiting body or mycelium and contain high levels of beta-glucans and related polysaccharides (crude hot-water extracts typically contain around 30% soluble polysaccharides, compared to 6-8% in the whole mushroom).
- Ethanolic (alcohol) extracts or tinctures – These contain higher levels of triterpenoid compounds but low levels of polysaccharides as the ethanol tends to precipitate the polysaccharides from solution. In some supplements they are combined with hot-water extracts to deliver high concentrations of both polysaccharides and triterpenes.

In general there are no more contraindications to taking mushroom supplements than there are to eating mushrooms (like them they should be avoided by those with an allergy to mushrooms) and all ages can benefit from them, including children and the elderly.

Contrary to popular belief they do not promote the growth of other fungi (quite the opposite) and are perfectly safe for those suffering from candida or other fungal conditions (*see box*).

Even animals can benefit from them and often respond well to mushroom supplementation in conditions including: cancer, allergies and respiratory problems.

Mushrooms and Candida

There is no truth in the widely disseminated view that mushrooms need to be avoided by those suffering from candida or other fungal conditions. Indeed, in many ways they are an ideal food in such cases as:

- They do not contain the types of sugars and refined carbohydrates that can stimulate candidal growth (mushroom polysaccharides are predominantly joined by beta-linkages that we cannot digest – hence their lack of sweetness).
- They increase the effectiveness of the immune system's response to candida and other fungi, as well as to cancer cells, virally infected cells and bacteria.
- They are a rich source of anti-fungal compounds – just as animals in the wild have to compete with each other for food, so mushrooms and other fungi have to compete with each other and with other micro-organisms for food. To help them do this fungi have evolved to produce, as well as antibiotics such as penicillin, a wide range of anti-fungal compounds, including proteins, triterpenes and polysaccharides.

This combination of immune system support with high levels of anti-fungal compounds is responsible for the effectiveness of mushroom supplementation in helping control candidal overgrowth, as confirmed by:

- Traditional use – mushrooms have traditionally been used to treat candida-related conditions such as thrush.
- Research – as well as identifying anti-fungal compounds produced by mushrooms, research confirms the ability of mushroom supplements to reduce candidal overgrowth and protect against candida infection[9-11].
- Clinical experience – mushroom supplements show efficacy as part of anti-candida protocols.

As with the majority of food supplements, the benefits of mushroom supplements are greatest when taken away from food, either between meals or 30 minutes before a meal, ideally with a glass of water. However, where this is not possible, they can be taken with food and powders can be blended with juice, added to a smoothie, or, where the flavour needs to be disguised, taken with stronger-tasting foods, such as: chocolate ice cream, mashed banana or peanut butter.

There is some evidence that vitamin C can enhance the bioavailability of mushroom polysaccharides and for this reason some authorities recommend that it be taken together with mushroom supplements.

As well as its undoubted health benefits, green tea may also offer synergistic benefits when taken together with mushrooms, with one Chinese study reporting an increased reduction in the risk of developing breast cancer among women who both consumed mushrooms and drank green tea on a regular basis[12].

Ten Medicinal Mushrooms

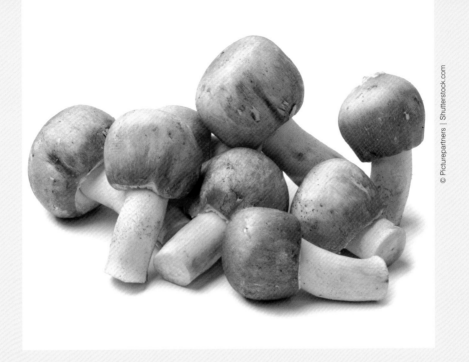

Almond Mushroom (Royal Sun Agaric)

Agaricus subrufescens (also known as *Agaricus blazei Murrill* and *Agaricus brasiliensis* – see ref.13 for discussion of its name)

Almond Mushroom grows widely, including in Europe and North America and derives its name from its somewhat sweet flavour and taste of almonds.

Main active components – As with all mushrooms, polysaccharides play a major role in Almond Mushroom's immunological activity, along with sterols and lipids, which in the closely related *Agaricus bisporus* have shown anti-aromatase activity[14].

Traditional use – Interest in Almond Mushroom's health benefits stems from reports linking its consumption with unusual longevity among inhabitants of Brazil's Piedade region.

Main Health Benefits

Cancer – A number of studies have been published reporting significant health benefits of Almond Mushroom for cancer patients.

In one study, increased NK cell activity was seen from supplementation with 3g/day of extract[15], while, in another, increased NK-cell activity and reduced chemotherapy-related side effects (reduced appetite, alopecia and general weakness) were reported from supplementation with Almond Mushroom polysaccharide extract in 100 cervical, ovarian, and endometrial cancer patients[16].

The ability of Almond Mushroom extract to help reduce side effects and improve treatment outcomes has also been reported in patients with acute non-lymphocytic leukaemia and advanced alimentary tract tumours[17], while improved metabolism and blood-pressure were seen in patients with colorectal cancer after surgery[18].

Hepatitis – As well as showing hepatoprotective properties in animal models, polysaccharide-rich hot-water extracts of Almond Mushroom have been investigated for their ability to support chronic hepatitis patients (B and C), with improvements in symptoms and reduction in liver enzymes reported from an intake of 1.5g/day[19].

Diabetes – Reductions in glucose levels have been reported in animal models of diabetes and supplementation with 1.5g/day of Almond Mushroom hot-water extract has also been reported to improve insulin resistance in type 2 diabetes in one randomized, double-blind, placebo-controlled clinical trial[14].

Notes – While traditional evidence points to benefits of the whole mushroom as a dietary component, clinical studies have focussed on polysaccharide-rich extracts.

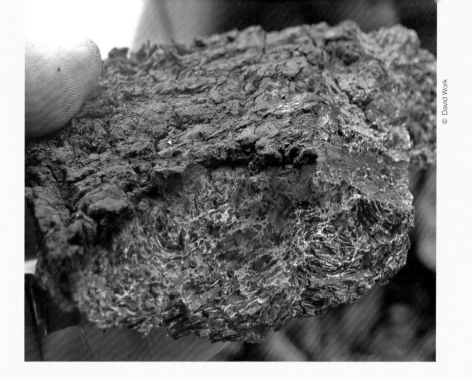

Chaga

Inonotus obliquus

Chaga grows widely in the forests of northern Europe, Asia and North America, forming a sterile growth or 'conk' with a typical burnt appearance that has led to it being known as the 'cinder-conk'.

Main active components – Unusually among medicinal mushrooms, Chaga's most important components are derived from the bark of the host birch trees on which it grows. Chief among these are a large number of betulinic acid derivatives and melano-glucan complexes.

Traditional use – Revered as a folk medicine, especially among the peoples of eastern Russia, Chaga has traditionally been boiled to make a tea, which is drunk to treat a range of conditions, including: cancers, viral and bacterial infections and gastro-intestinal disorders[20,21].

Main Health Benefits

Cancer – Betulinic acid shows wide-ranging anti-cancer activity, including against: leukaemia, malignant brain and peripheral nervous system cancers for which mushroom polysaccharide-based supplements show limited benefit[22].

As with other mushrooms, Chaga's polysaccharide components also show strong immune-modulating activity and this combination of mushroom polysaccharides with host-derived betulinic acid contributes to Chaga's traditional use in cancer treatment, including for: inoperable breast, lip, gastric, parotid, lung, skin, colorectal cancer and Hodgkin lymphoma[20].

Digestive disorders – Melano-glucan complexes have wide anti-microbial activity and Chaga has traditionally been used as an internal cleanser with Befungin, an alcohol extract of Chaga, licensed in Russia for the treatment of stomach and intestinal disorders[20].

Psoriasis – Several anecdotal reports indicate benefit of Chaga for psoriasis and this is supported by a Russian study on 50 psoriasis patients, which reported a 76% cure rate, with improvement in a further 16% of cases. The same study reported that it typically took 9-12 weeks for improvement to become apparent[23].

Notes – Chaga supplements need to be made from wild-harvested Chaga if they are to contain the main active components derived from the bark of the host birch trees.

Although most traditional use is based on hot-water extracts (teas), the triterpenoid betulinic acid derivatives (although not the polysaccharides) are more soluble in alcohol and for this reason tinctures or other alcohol-based extracts are sometimes used, either on their own or in combination with polysaccharide-rich hot-water extracts.

Traditionally around 5g of Chaga would be ground and boiled to make a tea, while the recommended daily dose of Befungin is 1tsp, three times a day and for extracts 1-3g/day.

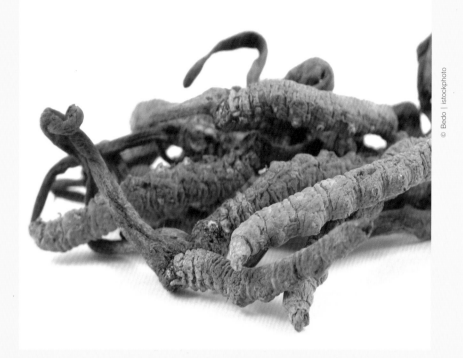

Cordyceps

Cordyceps species (see notes)

The Cordyceps species used medicinally have traditionally been found growing on the larvae of moths and it used to be thought that they were parasitic. However, it has also been suggested that they have a symbiotic relationship with their hosts, helping them thrive in extreme environments, such as the high Tibetan plateau, and only converting to their fruiting form on the death of the host insect[24].

Main active components – The ability of Cordyceps to increase metabolic efficiency and promote adaptation to harsh environments is largely due to the nucleoside derivatives (cordycepin, etc.) that it produces, which are also responsible for many of its unique health-promoting properties. In addition, polysaccharide fractions have shown significant immunomodulatory activity.

Traditional use – Because of its rarity, Cordyceps was traditionally restricted to the few who could afford it. Its main uses were in the treatment of asthma and erectile dysfunction, and as a tonic for the elderly and those recovering from long illness.

Main Health Benefits

Energy – In the same way that Cordyceps species help their hosts survive in oxygen-poor environments, Cordyceps-based products are used to enhance athletic performance and endurance by increasing the efficiency of energy metabolism.

Studies in healthy elderly subjects using Cs-4 (see below – 3g/day) showed significant increases in aerobic capacity and resistance to fatigue, while other research has shown increases in energy output and oxygen capacity in sedentary humans taking *C. sinensis* and increased endurance in animals given *C. militaris*[25,26].

Asthma/COPD – As well as increasing efficiency of energy metabolism, Cordyceps provides valuable support for those, including children, with impaired lung function from conditions such as asthma and COPD, based on an adult dose of 3g/day[24].

Anti-viral – The nucleoside analogues found in *C. militaris* and hybridized cordyceps species function as reverse transcriptase inhibitors, inhibiting viral replication. At the same time, cordyceps' polysaccharides have been shown to enhance the immune response to viral infections[24].

Cancer – Because of its combination of immune-modulating polysaccharides and nucleoside derivatives, many practitioners consider Cordyceps to be one of the most useful mushrooms for helping improve treatment outcomes in cancer, with cordycepin reported to induce apoptosis (cancer cell death) in multiple cancer cell lines, including: oral, colorectal, bladder, leukaemia, melanoma, multiple myeloma, breast and prostate (see notes).

Diabetes – Cordyceps provides useful support for cases of diabetes, with actions including:

- Triggering release of insulin
- Increasing hepatic glucokinase
- Increasing sensitivity of cells to insulin

Again, cordycepin and related nucleoside derivatives appear to play a key role in cordyceps' anti-diabetic action and cordycepin has also been shown to suppress the chronic low-grade inflammation associated with diabetes[27, 28].

Infertility – In addition to its traditional use for improving libido and treating erectile dysfunction, Cordyceps can be beneficial for both male and female infertility, with increases in steroid hormone production and improvements in testes morphology, sperm quantity and quality at a dose of 3-4.5g/day[29-31].

Kidney protective – The traditional use of Cordyceps to support the kidneys is backed-up by reports of improved kidney function in patients with chronic renal failure and speedier recovery in patients with antibiotic-induced kidney damage[24].

Hepatoprotective – Cordyceps can be a beneficial supplement for those suffering from impaired liver function, with inhibition of fibrosis and reductions in liver enzymes reported for liver conditions, including hepatitis and liver steatosis (fatty liver)[32].

Notes – Nowadays the Cordyceps available in supplement form is almost exclusively sourced from commercially cultivated material, dramatically increasing its availability, lowering its cost and making it suitable for vegetarians and vegans.

The move to cultivated material has led to a number of different Cordyceps products being available:

- *Cordyceps sinensis* – Strains of wild-harvested Cordyceps that have then been cultivated on grain-based substrates (solid fermentation / mycelial biomass technology).
- *Cordyceps militaris* – *C. militaris* has long been a common substitute for *C. sinensis* and, as *C. militaris* contains higher levels of cordycepin than *C. sinensis*, it may even be that it is at least partially responsible for the reverence in which *C. sinensis* has traditionally been held. Now artificially cultivated and harvested as fruiting bodies, as well as by solid fermentation / mycelial biomass technology. Sometimes called Cordyceps Flowers and known in Chinese as Yong Chong Cao.
- Cs-4 – Not strictly Cordyceps, Cs-4 has been identified as *Paecilomyces hepiali*, an organism isolated from wild *C. sinensis* specimens by China's Academy of Sciences and selected for ease of cultivation by large-scale liquid fermentation technology.

Although most studies have used 3.0 or 4.5g/day, supplementation of 1.5g/day can provide useful support for long term use.

Because Cordyceps has been shown to increase levels of male and female sex hormones, it may not be appropriate for those suffering from hormone dependent cancers (prostate and breast) and its hypoglycemic properties mean that it should be used with caution by those taking insulin.

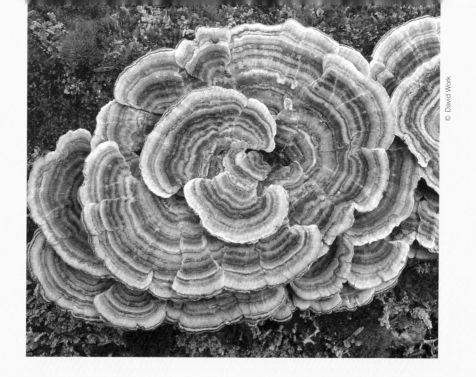

Coriolus

Trametes versicolor (formerly known as *Coriolus versicolor*)

This common woodland mushroom is the most widely researched of all the medicinal mushrooms. It is the source of the major pharmaceutical drugs: PSK (Krestin) and PSP, which are licensed in Japan and China respectively for use in cancer treatment, with annual sales of several hundred million US$.

Main active components – Like most mushroom polysaccharide extracts, both PSK and PSP are proteoglycans (polysaccharides with attached protein groups).

Traditional use – Coriolus is used in traditional Chinese medicine to strengthen the immune system, treat lung and urinary tract infections, tumours and liver disorders.

Main Health Benefits

Cancer – The Coriolus extracts PSP and PSK are routinely used alongside conventional treatment in the Far East, typically at 3g/day, with over 40 randomized controlled trials confirming benefit for a range of cancers, including: stomach cancer, colorectal cancer, lung cancer (NSCLC), oesophageal cancer, nasopharyngeal cancer, breast cancer and cervical/uterine cancer.

Reported benefits include increases in 2, 5 and 15 year survival, as well as reduced side-effects from conventional treatment[33-35].

Anti-viral – Coriolus' ability to support healthy immune function means that it is also an excellent supplement for chronic viral conditions[36], including:

Herpes – Coriolus has been shown to inactivate Herpes Simplex Virus (HSV) in a dose-dependent manner and clinically is seen to reduce the frequency of HSV outbreaks.

HIV – *In-vitro* studies show anti-HIV activity of Coriolus extracts and clinical reports indicate improvement in HIV patients' immune status from Coriolus mycelial biomass supplementation.

Chronic Fatigue Syndrome (CFS/ME) – Many cases of CFS are associated with high viral levels and Coriolus mycelial biomass (1.5-3g/day) has been shown to provide effective support, helping improve quality of life scores, lower viral levels and improve immune parameters, including increased NK cell activity[37].

Anti-fungal – Coriolus extracts have a pronounced protective effect against lethal infection with Candida albicans in mice[11].

Notes – Clinical trials using high concentration extracts, such as PSK and PSP, are mostly at a dose of 3g/day. Research with mycelial biomass products shows benefit at the same supplementation level.

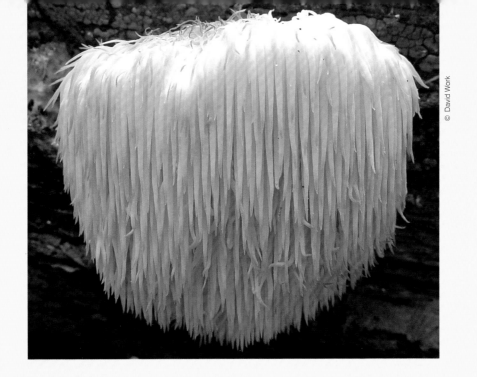

© David Work

Lion's Mane (Hedgehog/Monkey-head Mushroom)
Hericium erinaceus

Growing on hardwood trees in temperate forests across the northern hemisphere, Lion's Mane is a delicious culinary mushroom with a growing reputation as a medicinal mushroom.

Main active components – Lion's Mane's unique properties are due to two families of compounds that it produces: the erinacines and hericenones, which, as well as having strong anti-bacterial activity, help stimulate the generation of Nerve Growth Factor (NGF).

Traditional use – Traditional use of Lion's Mane emphasises its anti-microbial and immunonological activity, with indications including gastric and duodenal ulcers, chronic gastritis, gastric and oesophageal cancer.

Main Health Benefits

Dementia/Alzheimer's disease – Patients with dementia have lower than normal levels of NGF and the ability of Lion's Mane's erinacines and hericenones to increase production of NGF makes it a particularly beneficial supplement for individuals with mild dementia.

Positive results have been reported in two small-scale clinical studies (using 3g/day in one study and 2g/day in the other), with improvements in: functional capacity (understanding, communication, memory etc.), functional independence scores (eating, dressing, walking etc.) and cognitive function[38,39].

Neuropathy – NGF also plays an important role in pain sensitivity and low NGF levels have been linked to neuropathy in both animal and *in-vitro* studies. Clinically Lion's Mane is seen to be beneficial for neuropathy from a variety of causes, including multiple sclerosis[40,41].

Nerve damage – Lion's Mane is also beneficial in many cases of nerve damage from traumatic injury, helping promote faster regrowth, mirroring the results seen from animal studies[42].

Menopausal syndrome – Some of the compounds that help generate NGF have been shown to have a calming effect and this may account for the clinically observed benefit of Lion's Mane for menopausal syndrome with patients reporting significant improvements in sleep-disturbance, anxiety and hot flushes (hot flashes)[43].

Anti-bacterial – The erinacines and hericenones are produced by Lion's Mane for their potent anti-microbial activity and effectiveness against MRSA has been reported from both laboratory tests and clinical studies[44,45].

Notes – Although clinical trials have used dried fruiting body at a dose of 2-5g/day, it is probable that mycelial mycelial biomass may offer similar benefits at lower supplementation levels.

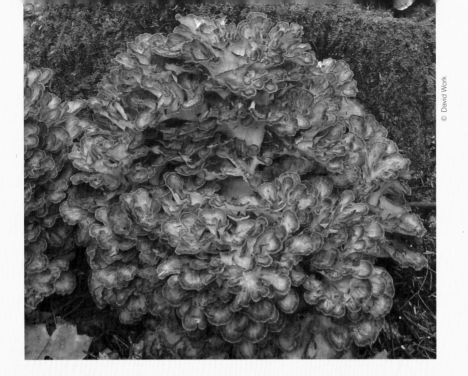

© David Work

Maitake

Grifola frondosa

Maitake and the closely related Umbrella Polypore (*Polyporus umbellatus*) are both delicious gourmet mushrooms, as well as being highly regarded for their health benefits. Indeed, the name 'Maitake' means 'Dancing Mushroom' in Japanese, indicating people's joy at finding it!

Main active components – Polysaccharides are the principal active components in Maitake, with several fractions, including: D-fraction and MD-fraction, showing strong immunological activity[46,47].

Traditional use – Most traditional sources do not mention Maitake and it appears that it was often not differentiated from Umbrella Polypore (also known as *Grifola umbellata*), of which it is said that 'long term use makes one feel happy and vigorous and look younger'.

Main Health Benefits

Cancer – Impressive results have been reported from the use of Maitake polysaccharide extracts, or combinations of polysaccharide extracts and fruiting body, with one study using 40-100mg MD-fraction and 4-6g powdered fruiting body reporting cancer regression or significant symptom improvement in 58% of liver cancer patients, 68% of breast cancer patients and 62% of lung cancer patients.

Similar results have been reported using combinations of D-fraction and powdered fruiting body and improvements in immune-competent cell activities have also been reported when taken in conjunction with chemotherapy[48,49].

Polysaccharide extracts of Umbrella Polypore are also licensed as anti-cancer agents in China, with improved treatment outcomes and quality of life indicators in a number of cancers, including: lung, liver, leukaemia, bladder, nose and throat[50].

Diabetes – Several studies report significant improvement in blood sugar levels in type II diabetes patients from using purified Maitake polysaccharides. Positive results have also been reported from inclusion of crude Maitake powder in the diet of diabetic animal models (20% of food, or 1g/day in a mouse model)[51,52].

Polycystic Ovary Syndrome (PCOS) – In the majority of cases, PCOS is associated with some level of insulin resistance and Maitake polysaccharide extracts also show promise as agents for helping address this condition[53].

In one Japanese study, ovulation was observed in 20 of the 26 women given a Maitake polysaccharide extract and 6 of 8 women who failed to ovulate after being treated with clomiphene citrate did so after being given the polysaccharide extract. In addition, all 3 women who expressed an interest in becoming pregnant were able to do so[54].

Notes – Polysaccharide extracts or combinations of extract and fruiting body have been favoured clinically at doses of 3-6g/day.

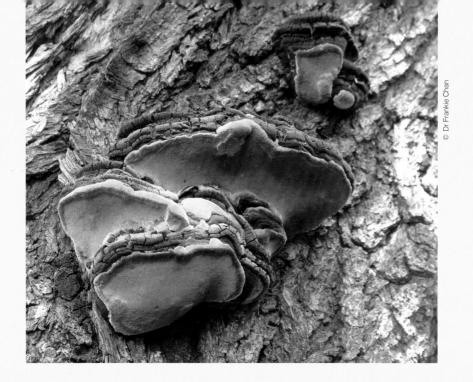

Mesima

Phellinus linteus

Mesima is a highly sought after traditional remedy in Korea and is also common in south-east Asia and the southern United States.

Main active components – Research has focussed on hot-water proteoglycan extracts. However, polyphenols and triterpenoid compounds are also believed to contribute to the health benefits of Mesima and related Phellinus species[55-57].

Traditional use – In Korea, Mesima is drunk as a tea and is believed to be responsible for a number of cases of spontaneous recovery from various cancers, including prostate and liver cancer. In the official Chinese Pharmacopoeia it is also indicated for: diabetes, HIV, angina, leucorrhoea, diarrhoea and accelerated wound healing.

Main Health Benefits

Cancer – As well as multiple reports of spontaneous remission, laboratory studies show Mesima extracts to have exceptionally high immunological activity and a range of anti-cancer effects against different cancer cell lines, including lung, breast and prostate cancer[58,59].

Mesima extracts have also been shown to enhance the efficacy of existing chemotherapeutic agents[60].

Benign Prostatic Hyperplasia (BPH) – Hot-water extract of Mesima has shown benefit in reducing BPH in animal models[61].

Auto-immune conditions – As well as its traditional use for cancer support, Mesima shows considerable promise in the management of a number of auto-immune conditions, including:

Infertility – In cases where infertility is due to elevated cytokine and NK cell levels, Mesima has been found to be effective in helping reduce these, with 23 of 26 women showing improvement in one study[62].

Rheumatoid arthritis – Several animal studies confirm benefits for rheumatoid arthritis from polysaccharide and proteoglycan extracts of Mesima and related species, with reductions in inflammation and inflammatory immune markers[63,64].

Allergies – Studies also show benefits of Mesima polysaccharide extracts for allergies, with reports that they help re-balance immune responses and inhibit histamine release in cases of allergic reaction[65].

Notes – While most research has focussed on polysaccharide extracts, studies on Mesima's use for infertility have used mycelial biomass at 3g/day.

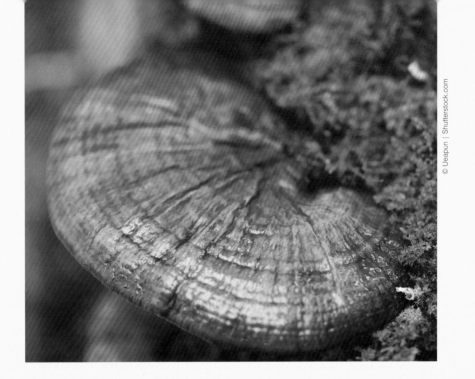

Reishi

Ganoderma lucidum

Revered by emperors and sages alike, and associated in oriental culture with happiness, health and good fortune, Reishi's extensive health benefits have led to it being known as the 'Mushroom of Immortality' or '10,000 Year Mushroom' (Mannentake), with annual sales of over US$2.5 billion.

Although primarily cultivated in China and east Asia, Reishi species grow widely throughout Europe and North America, with the original description of *Ganoderma lucidum* being based on material collected in London, U.K. in 1781.

Main active components – Reishi's wide-ranging health benefits are due to its combination of highly active immune-modulating poly-saccharides and over 130 triterpenoid compounds (primarily ganoderic and lucidenic acids), with actions including: anti-inflammatory, anti-histamine, sedative, anti-hypertensive and anti-cancer[66].

Traditional use – Reishi has traditionally been associated with the Taoist quest for immortality, as well as being used to treat a range of health conditions, including: cancer, heart disease and bronchitis.

Main Health Benefits

Cancer – Reishi has a long history of use in cancer treatment with many reports of spontaneous remission[67].

Although both polysaccharides and triterpenes contribute to Reishi's anti-cancer action, clinical trials have focussed exclusively the more easily characterised polysaccharide extracts, with a recent review of 5 randomised controlled trials indicating that patients given Reishi polysaccharide extracts were 1.27 times more likely to respond positively to chemo/radiotherapy than those without[68].

At the same time, Reishi's triterpenes also show extensive anti-cancer activity, inhibiting cancer cell growth, inducing apoptosis (cell death) and, in the case of prostate cancer cells, blocking androgen receptors[69].

Allergies – Reishi's combination of high immuno-modulatory activity with strong anti-inflammatory and anti-histamine activity make it a uniquely suitable supplement for those suffering from allergies such as hayfever (allergic rhinitis)[70].

By addressing both the underlying immune imbalance that predisposes the body to overreacting to pollen or other allergens, as well as the histamine-mediated inflammatory responses that result, it can be used to both help alleviate the symptoms and prevent their development.

Auto-immune disease – Reishi's combination of immunomodulatory and anti-inflammatory action also makes it a useful supplement for a range of inflammatory auto-immune conditions, such as rheumatoid arthritis, psoriasis or ulcerative colitis.

Insomnia/anxiety – The traditional name 'spirit mushroom' points to the sedative action of Reishi's triterpenoid components. Improvements in sleep patterns are one of the most commonly reported effects of Reishi supplementation and it is frequently prescribed for this purpose[71].

Liver disease – Reishi has long been a popular traditional treatment for liver diseases and demonstrates wide hepatoprotective properties, including:
- Protection from chemical toxicity
- Inhibition of liver fibrosis
- Normalisation of liver enzymes
- Reduction in inflammation

Cardiovascular health – Traditionally used in the treatment of heart disease, Reishi has been shown to support cardiovascular health through cholesterol-lowering, blood-pressure lowering and anti-coagulant effects, with improvements in ECG, chest pain, palpitations and shortness of breath reported in one randomized, double-blind, multi-centred study using a polysaccharide extract at 5.4g/day[72].

Respiratory health – As well as its benefits for cardiovascular health, Reishi has traditionally been used to treat bronchitis, with older patients showing particular benefit.

Its anti-allergic properties mean that it is helpful for allergic asthma, while Chinese studies also report alleviation of altitude sickness[73].

Notes – Classically differentiated according to six different colours, today virtually all cultivated Reishi is Red Reishi, with the term Duanwood Red Reishi sometimes being used to refer to cultivation on whole logs, as opposed to cultivation on 'logs' made of compressed sawdust.

Reishi's uniquely broad health benefits are due to its combination of immune-modulating, water-soluble polysaccharides and anti-inflammatory triterpenes, which are poorly water-soluble.

In order to deliver high levels of both polysaccharides and triterpenes, supplements may combine both polysaccharide-rich hot-water and triterpene-rich ethanolic (alcohol-based) extracts. Alternatively, some supplements use Reishi spores, which also contain high levels of triterpenes, with oil-based spore extracts containing up to 30%.

Supplementation levels of Reishi products can vary considerably owing to the range of product types available. Most trials using polysaccharide extract have been at 5.4g/day, while daily consumption of pure Reishi powder can be considerably higher. Products combining Reishi polysaccharides and triterpenes typically have dosage ranges of 1-3g/day, Reishi sporoderm-broken spore products 3-5g/day and Reishi spore oil extracts 500-1,500mg/day.

Reishi's triterpenes have been reported to have anti-coagulant properties and supplements containing high levels should be used with caution by those on blood-thinning medication.

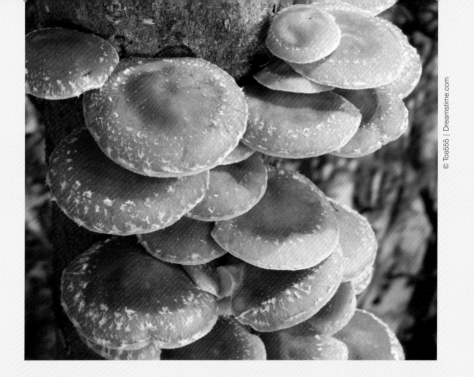

Shiitake

Lentinula edodes (formerly called *Lentinus edodes*)

Shiitake is the second most widely cultivated mushroom, after the common button mushroom. It combines an excellent nutritional profile and exceptional culinary properties with significant health benefits and is the source of Lentinan, a polysaccharide extract licensed in Japan for use in the treatment of stomach cancer.

Like other mushrooms, fresh Shiitake can be a useful source of vitamin D2, providing it is exposed to sunlight or UV light either before or after harvesting.

Principle active compounds – As well as Lentinan and other poly-saccharides, Shiitake produces a number of anti-microbial compounds, including eritadenine, which has been shown to help lower blood cholesterol levels[74].

Traditional use – Although traditionally used principally as a culinary mushroom, Shiitake's anti-cancer properties have been extensively researched in Japan since the 1960s.

Main Health Benefits

Cancer – Lentinan has been shown to offer a significant advantage over chemotherapy alone in terms of survival for patients with advanced gastric cancer, with additional trials reporting increased survival, reduced chemotherapy-related side effects and improved quality of life in patients with: colorectal, liver, breast and metastatic prostate cancer[75,76].

Although clinical trials with Shiitake have almost exclusively used Lentinan delivered by injection, recent research indicates that it is also orally bioavailable[77].

Cholesterol control – Shiitake's eritadenine content makes it a useful dietary supplement for those seeking to control their cholesterol levels, with two small-scale clinical studies reporting decreases in total cholesterol and triglycerides from consumption of Shiitake (9g/day dried in one and 90g/day fresh in another)[74].

Anti-viral – As with other mushrooms rich in immunologically active polysaccharides, Shiitake's ability to strengthen immune function helps improve immune response to a range of viral conditions, including:
- Hepatitis
- Influenza
- HIV

Notes – Because eritadenine's cholesterol lowering action differs from that of prescription statins, or natural sources of statins such as Red Yeast Rice (*Monascus purpureus*), Shiitake can be a particularly useful dietary supplement for those already taking statins or for whom they are unsuitable due to the level of side-effects.

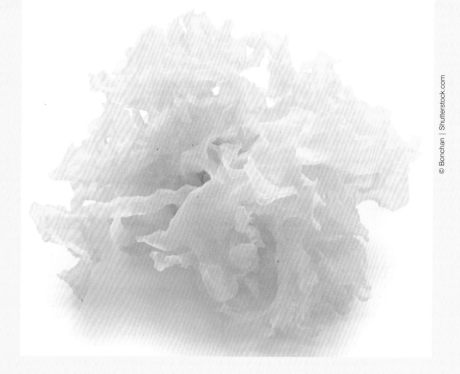

Snow Fungus

Tremella fuciformis

Snow Fungus is an excellent mushroom for health maintenance and in its dried form is a popular ingredient in oriental cuisine, prized for its translucent appearance and crunchy texture.

Main active components – Snow Fungus contains high levels of immunologically active polysaccharides which are structurally distinct from those found in most other medicinal mushrooms and are the key components responsible for its health benefits[78].

Traditional use – In traditional Chinese medicine, Snow Fungus is listed in the highest category of herbs, with indications including:
  • Clearing heat and moistening dryness
  • Nourishing the brain and enhancing beauty

Main Health Benefits

Cardiovascular health – Snow Fungus is eaten to help prevent atherosclerosis in Japan and provides support for the cardiovascular system by[79]:

- Helping maintain the health of blood-vessel walls
- Helping prevent clots and enhance circulation
- Lowering cholesterol

In this respect its actions are similar to the closely related Wood Ear (*Auricularia auricula*/*Auricularia polytricha*).

Anti-ageing – As well as their benefits for the cardiovascular system, Snow Fungus' polysaccharides combine a number of other anti-ageing properties[80]:

- Increasing the superoxide dismutase activity of the brain and liver.
- Promoting nerve growth
- Assisting with improving learning and reducing memory deficits
- Supporting skin-health, including as a moisturizing agent in cosmetic preparations
- Anti-inflammatory

Protection from radiation – Snow Fungus polysaccharide-based products are used in China to help patients undergoing radiotherapy by[78]:

- Supporting the immune system
- Maintaining white blood cell counts
- Alleviating skin dryness and redness

Notes – While 5-10g/day of dried Snow Fungus or 1-2g/day of polysaccharide extract are beneficial for general health maintenance, studies on radiation exposure have used 3-5g/day of polysaccharide extract.

Health Benefits of Medicinal Mushrooms

The following is a summary of the main health areas and conditions for which mushrooms show benefit.

The fact that a particular mushroom or mushrooms is listed against a given condition does not mean that other mushrooms will not be of benefit, just that the evidence for them is not as strong. Where the benefits of mushrooms for a given condition are due to the immune-modulating activity of the beta-glucans and related polysaccharide components found in all species, and there is evidence indicating benefit for multiple mushrooms, no single mushroom is specified.

Supplementation levels will vary according to the individual and the form in which the mushroom is taken. For discussion of different dosage forms the reader is referred to the Introduction and for typical supplementation levels to the sections on each mushroom.

As always, those with any medical condition should seek the advice of an appropriately qualified healthcare practitioner and those taking prescription medication should consult their prescriber before making any changes.

Alzheimer's disease – see Dementia

Anxiety – see Insomnia/Anxiety

Asthma

Cordyceps is widely used to support lung function, including in conditions such as asthma and COPD, with one study reporting an 81.3% symptom reduction within an average of 5 days[24].

Where asthma is primarily triggered by exposure to allergens, Reishi can be particularly effective, either on its own or in combination with Cordyceps, by virtue of its triterpenoid components, which have strong anti-inflammatory and anti-histamine activity.

Cordyceps and/or Reishi

Bacterial infection

Many mushrooms, like other fungi, produce antibiotic compounds in order to help them compete for resources in their natural habitat and the diverse array of natural antibiotics they produce accounts for their widespread anti-bacterial activity.

In particular, the erinacines and hericenones produced by Lion's Mane show strong action against a range of bacteria, including MRSA and Helicobacter pylori, the bacteria responsible for most gastric ulcers[44,45].

Lion's Mane

Benign Prostatic Hyperplasia (BPH)

Although there have as yet been no clinical studies, triterpenoid compounds from Reishi have a marked anti-androgenic effect and have been shown to reduce testosterone-induced growth of the prostate in animal studies[81].

At the same time, polysaccharide-rich extracts from Mesima have been reported to reduce cellular proliferation in animal models of BPH[61].

Reishi and/or Mesima

Cancer

Because of their ability to help restore healthy immune function (see Introduction), mushrooms can be a beneficial food for cancer patients and for those seeking to avoid cancer, with a large number of studies showing improvement in treatment outcomes and reduction in side-effects from combining mushroom supplements with conventional treatment, as well as several studies showing a link between increased mushroom consumption and reduced risk of developing cancer[1,2,82].

The key immune-modulating polysaccharides are present in all mushrooms as part of the mushroom cell-wall and anti-cancer activity has been demonstrated for extracts from over 650 mushrooms. However, clinical research has tended to focus on a smaller number of mushrooms from which proprietary extracts have been developed.

Clinical trials using extracts of these mushrooms alongside conventional cancer therapies have demonstrated increased survival for a range of solid tumours, with lower levels of evidence for blood-based cancers such as leukaemia.

Multiple studies have also demonstrated a reduced level of side-effects from conventional cancer treatment, including reductions in nausea and fatigue associated with chemotherapy and maintenance of white blood cell counts and other immune parameters during both radiotherapy and chemotherapy.

The following notes on individual cancers are based where possible on clinical research. However, research is inevitably biased towards the mushrooms used to produce the products manufactured by the companies paying for the research and in cases where the main active component is polysaccharide-based it is reasonable to assume that other mushrooms may show similar effects.

Supplementation levels will vary considerably depending on the nature of the supplement and the stage of treatment, with higher levels usually appropriate to provide support during active treatment and lower levels during maintenance and recovery phases. In addition, there is some evidence that combining different mushrooms can enhance their effectiveness and a number of mushroom supplement combinations are available.

Typical Supplementation Levels
- *Support during treatment – 3-6g/day (some practitioners recommend higher levels, particularly for non-extract-based products)*
- *Maintenance – 1-3g/day*

Bladder cancer – Maitake shows high levels of activity against bladder cancer cell lines and extracts from the closely related Umbrella Polypore are used alongside conventional therapy in the treatment of bladder cancer in China.

Brain cancer – Although there have been no published clinical trials, betulinic acid, found in wild-harvested Chaga, has been shown to inhibit growth of various brain cancer cell lines *in-vitro* and supplementation with Maitake has been reported to produce improvement in some cases.

Breast cancer – Two epidemiological studies have reported reduced rates of breast cancer in women who regularly consume mushrooms, with one of the studies reporting a greater effect in post-menopausal women[12,83]. At the same time, clinical trials with a number of mushrooms have reported benefits in the treatment of breast cancer, including: Coriolus, Maitake and Almond Mushroom.

Cervical cancer – Almond Mushroom extract has been reported to enhance immune parameters and reduce side effects in patients with cervical cancer undergoing chemotherapy, while Coriolus mycelial biomass increased clearance rates in women with LSIL (see HPV)[16,84].

Colorectal cancer – A number of clinical trials in Japan showed clear benefit from supplementation with 3g/day Coriolus extract in improving both survival and disease-free survival in cases of curatively resected colorectal cancer and research on extracts of Reishi and Shiitake has also produced positive results[85,86].

Leukaemia – Although a number of *in-vitro* studies have shown activity of extracts from different mushrooms to be effective in inducing apoptosis (cell death) in leukaemia cells and isolated clinical reports indicate possible benefit, clinical trials with Coriolus extract failed to show a statistically significant improvement in treatment outcomes.

Liver cancer – Supplementation with Maitake has been reported to be beneficial for patents with liver cancer, while *in-vitro* and animal studies indicate benefit from extracts of other mushrooms, including Almond Mushroom, Shiitake, Reishi and Cordyceps.

Lung cancer – Extracts from both Coriolus and Maitake have been reported to be beneficial in cases of lung cancer with one trial using an extract of Coriolus (3g every other day) reporting a nearly 5-fold increase in survival after 5 years[87].

Lymphoma – Clinical data is so far lacking but animal and *in-vitro* studies support reports of benefit and reduction in symptoms from conventional treatment.

Multiple myeloma – *In-vitro* research has indicated that Cordyceps may be of benefit in cases of multiple myeloma, with cordycepin being shown to induce cell death in multiple myeloma cells[88].

Ovarian cancer – As with cervical and endometrial cancer, Almond Mushroom extract has been reported to enhance immune parameters and reduce side-effects in patients undergoing conventional treatment[16].

Pancreatic cancer – Individual reports indicate that there may be benefit from combining mushroom extracts with conventional treatment, while unpublished research from China points to increased survival duration from consumption of Reishi extract (combined fruiting body, mycelium and spore extracts) at a dose of 12g/day[89].

Prostate cancer – Several mushrooms have been shown to be beneficial for prostate cancer with Reishi often preferred because of its combination of immune modulating polysaccharides and anti-androgenic triterpenes[90].

Skin cancer – Studies have shown positive results from extracts of Maitake, Cordyceps and Coriolus in animal models of skin cancer. However, to date there have been no clinical trials.

Stomach (Gastric) cancer – Extracts of both Coriolus (PSK, given orally) and Shiitake (Lentinan, given by injection) are licensed in Japan as adjuvant nutrition in the treatment of stomach cancer with extensive clinical trials confirming their benefit in this area.

Uterine cancer – Almond Mushroom extract has been reported to enhance immune parameters and reduce side-effects in patients undergoing conventional treatment[16].

Candida

Mushroom supplementation can play a valuable role in anti-candida protocols through its ability to increase the efficacy of the immune system's response to candida, as well as to other fungal pathogens (see introduction for further discussion). Almond Mushroom, Coriolus and Shiitake all show efficacy in this regard and it is likely that further research would confirm similar benefits for other mushrooms[9-11].

Almond Mushroom/Coriolus/Shiitake

Cardiovascular health

Reishi and Snow Fungus in particular show promise for supporting cardiovascular health, with actions including:
* Anti-oxidant
* Anti-inflammatory
* Cholesterol-lowering
* Anti-thrombotic

A polysaccharide extract from Reishi has been reported to reduce chest pain, palpitations and shortness of breath in one clinical study, while Snow Fungus polysaccharides have been shown to help protect the cells lining the blood vessels, damage to which is an important contributory factor in the development of cardiovascular disease[72,79].

Reishi and/or Snow Fungus

Crohn's disease – See Inflammatory bowel disease

Chronic Fatigue Syndrome (CFS – M.E.)

Although the cause is not yet clear, CFS is typically accompanied by signs of a chronic pro-inflammatory immune state with high levels of pro-inflammatory cytokines (chemical messengers), low levels of NK cell activity and high viral counts.

Sufferers often find the immune-modulating action of mushroom polysaccharides helpful in restoring immune balance and clinical studies with Coriolus mycelial biomass confirm the potential of mushroom nutrition in this regard.

Coriolus

Colds / Flu
Individuals taking mushroom supplements on a regular basis typically report lowered incidences of colds and flu, and clinical studies indicate benefit for children suffering from recurrent respiratory tract infections[91].

Various Mushrooms

Dementia
Lion's Mane's ability to promote production of Nerve Growth Factor (low in dementia and Alzheimer's disease) makes it an ideal supplement for sufferers, especially in the early stages of the condition, with clinical studies confirming benefit, both from culinary consumption and from consumption as tablets[38,39].

Lion's Mane

Diabetes
As well as being an ideal food for those with diabetes with an excellent nutritional profile and low glycaemic index, several mushrooms have been shown to help control blood glucose levels in both human and animal studies, including: Cordyceps, Lion's Mane, Maitake, Reishi, Snow Fungus and Almond Mushroom; with Cordyceps and Maitake showing particular promise in this regard when used alongside appropriate dietary and lifestyle regimens.

Cordyceps and/or Maitake

Digestive health
Chaga has traditionally been used to support the digestive system and its combination of immune-modulating polysaccharides with anti-microbial triterpenes and melano-glucan complexes make it a particularly useful addition to protocols designed to address both inflammatory and infectious digestive disorders.

Chaga

Erectile dysfunction
Although not an instant 'pick-me-up', when taken on an ongoing basis Cordyceps can produce improvements in cases of erectile dysfunction, depending on the cause, in line with its traditional use for this indication[24].

Cordyceps

Fatigue
Where fatigue is due to physical exertion, or the demands of a hectic lifestyle, Cordyceps can help provide increased levels of energy. Unlike tonic herbs, such as ginseng, it does not provide an immediate boost and as with its use for erectile dysfunction it needs to be taken on an ongoing basis for its effects to be felt[24].

Where fatigue is a side effect of an underlying immune-deficient condition such as cancer or CFS mushroom supplementation often results in feelings of increased energy as immune balance improves.

Cordyceps/Various Mushrooms

Hayfever (Allergic rhinitis)
Reishi's combination of triterpenoid compounds with anti-inflammatory and anti-histamine activity and immune-modulating polysaccharides helps address both the symptoms and the underlying immune

imbalance responsible for hayfever and related allergic disorders. It is thus an ideal supplement for hayfever sufferers, showing benefit both for prevention and for alleviation of symptoms[70].

Reishi

Hepatitis
Clinical studies using several species of mushroom have shown positive results in cases of hepatitis (B and C) with Reishi, Cordyceps and Almond Mushroom showing particular promise.

Reishi/Cordyceps/Almond Mushroom

Herpes
As with hepatitis and other chronic viral conditions, herpes infections respond well to mushroom supplementation and although most research has focussed on Coriolus, it is likely that other mushrooms would show similar benefits.

Coriolus

High blood pressure (HBP)
Although animal studies have shown benefit for mushroom supplementation in high blood pressure models, in the absence of clinical trials their benefits in this area remain unproven.

Of the mushrooms that have potential in this area, Reishi's is thought to be the greatest, with several of its triterpenes showing ACE-inhibitory activity.

Reishi

High cholesterol
Beta-glucans from several sources including mushrooms have now

been shown to help with maintaining healthy cholesterol levels. In addition, several mushrooms are natural sources of lovastatin with Reishi mycelium having particularly high levels[92].

In cases where statin class compounds are not appropriate Shiitake combines the cholesterol-lowering beta-glucans with eritadenine, which helps the body control cholesterol levels through a different mechanism than that involved in the activity of statins and has been shown to be helpful in reducing cholesterol levels in clinical studies with daily consumption of 9g dried Shiitake producing a 10% reduction in cholesterol levels[75].

Shiitake

HIV

In common with other chronic viral conditions, mushroom supplements show benefit for maintaining immune competency in the face of HIV infection, with clinical reports focussing on polysaccharides from Coriolus and other mushrooms.

In addition, Cordyceps' nucleoside derivatives function as reverse transcriptase inhibitors, inhibiting viral replication and making Cordyceps a potentially important supplement for those suffering from HIV, while a number of triterpenoid compounds, including those found in Chaga and Reishi, show direct anti-HIV activity.

Various Mushrooms

HPV

Coriolus biomass supplementation has been shown to improve clearance of early stage cervical dysplasia (LSIL) and associated high-risk HPV strains, with 12 months supplementation at 3g/day increasing clearance from 50% to 91%[84].

Coriolus

Infertility – Female

As with male infertility, Cordyceps shows benefits for female infertility and is a widely used supplement in this regard.

Where infertility is due to immune imbalances, Mesima shows benefits for restoring normal NK cell and cytokine levels, while reports indicate that Maitake polysaccharide extracts can help where infertility is associated with Polycystic Ovary Syndrome[54,62].

Cordyceps and/or Mesima

Infertility – Male

Animal studies have shown Cordyceps supplementation to increase sperm quantity and quality, confirming clinical experience and supporting its traditional use in this area[24].

Cordyceps

Inflammatory bowel disease

Several animal studies show a protective effect from consumption of whole mushroom material and from supplementation with mushroom polysaccharide extracts in inflammatory bowel disease models.

Various Mushrooms

Insomnia /Anxiety

A number of Reishi's triterpenoid components show sedative activity and many people report improvements in sleep and reductions in anxiety from taking it. In addition, Lion's Mane often produces a pronounced calming effect and shows particular promise for menopause-related sleep disturbance.

Reishi and/or Lions Mane

Kidney health

Cordyceps has traditionally been used to strengthen the kidneys and adrenals and clinical studies have indicated benefit in cases of chronic renal failure and antibiotic-induced kidney damage[24].

Cordyceps

Liver health

Research on many mushrooms indicates widespread benefits for liver health, including protection from toxins and recovery from infection, while Cordyceps and Reishi have also been shown to: inhibit liver fibrosis, reduce liver inflammation and help normalize liver enzyme levels in cases of fatty liver (liver steatosis)[93, 94].

Cordyceps and/or Reishi

Menopausal syndrome

Although not included among its traditional indications, clinically I find that Lion's Mane gives significant relief to many women experiencing menopausal symptoms such as: hot flushes (hot flashes), anxiety and insomnia.

Lion's Mane

Nerve damage

Lion's Mane's ability to promote the production of nerve growth factor makes it an excellent mushroom for helping support recovery of damaged nerves, with clinical reports confirming results from *in-vitro* and animal studies[42].

Lion's Mane

Neuropathy

Together with its benefits for nerve damage, Lion's Mane also shows promise addressing conditions characterised by chronic neuropathy.

Lion's Mane

Polymyalgia rheumatica – See Rheumatoid arthritis

Polycystic Ovary Syndrome (PCOS)

As well as helping the insulin resistance often associated with PCOS, Maitake polysaccharide extracts show benefit in the management of PCOS itself, with one study reporting ovulation in 20 of 26 women given a Maitake polysaccharide extract, including 6 of 8 women who failed to ovulate after other treatments, and positive results in cases of PCOS-related infertility[54].

Maitake

Psoriasis

As with other autoimmune conditions, mushroom nutrition can be helpful in cases of psoriasis with one study using a Chaga extract reporting a 76% cure rate and clinical reports also indicating benefit from use of a Reishi extract-based product[23].

Chaga and/or Reishi

Rheumatoid arthritis

Mushroom nutrition can also play a useful role in strategies to treat other autoimmune conditions, including: rheumatoid arthritis, psoriatic arthritis and polymyalgia rheumatica.

Mesima appears particularly effective in this regard, as does Reishi, which also benefits from the anti-inflammatory properties of its ganoderic and lucidenic acids, making it particularly suitable for more active phases[63].

Reishi and/or Mesima

Smoking-related conditions
Snow Fungus combines several health benefits that make it a useful supplement for those who find it difficult to stop smoking, including:
- Supporting immune balance
- Promoting blood-vessel health
- Helping lower cholesterol
- Alleviating dry skin

Snow Fungus

Glossary

ACE Inhibitor – major category of blood pressure lowering drugs.

Anti-thrombotic – helping prevent the formation of blood clots.

Aromatase – an enzyme responsible for a key step in estrogen synthesis, inhibition of which significantly lowers estrogen levels.

Beta-glucan – the prototypical mushroom polysaccharide, composed of predominantly glucose units joined by beta linkages, which our digestive enzymes cannot break (unlike the alpha linkages that join the sugar units in starch molecules). In many cases mushrooms beta-glucans consist of a main chain of beta 1-3 linked sugar units, joined to side chains by beta 1-6 linkages and are referred to as 1-3, 1-6 beta-glucans.

Cervical dysplasia – abnormal cervical cells. Sometimes a precursor to the development of cervical cancer.

COPD – Chronic Obstructive Pulmonary Disease - another term for chronic bronchitis or emphysema, where the airways narrow over the course of time.

Cytokines – chemical messengers produced by immune cells.

ECG – Electrocardiogram - a technique to diagnose and measure abnormal rhythms of the heart.

Hepatic glucokinase – an important enzyme in the regulation of glucose metabolism.

Hepatoprotective – liver protective.

HPV – Human Papillomavirus – Over 120 strains of HPV are known and several have been implicated in different health conditions, including genital warts and cervical cancer.

Hypoglycemic – blood sugar lowering.

Immune-modulation – balancing the immune system, increasing depressed levels of immune activity and decreasing elevated immune responses.

Interferons – chemical messengers that help facilitate effective immune response to pathogens or tumours.

in-vitro – laboratory experiments that do not use animals.

LSIL – Low-grade Squamous Intraepithelial Lesions.

Metastasis – the spread of cancer to new areas of the body.

MRSA – Methicillin Resistant Staphylococcus Aureus - the 'Superbug'.

NK cells – Natural Killer cells – an important component in the immune system's response to pathogens and cancer.

NSCLC – Non-Small Cell Lung Cancer.

Nucleoside – the building blocks of DNA and RNA. Nucleoside analogues are molecules that resemble nucleosides but lack key functional group(s) and so act to block DNA/RNA replication.

Polysaccharides – molecules formed of a long chain of sugar units, often, in the case of mushroom polysaccharides, with bound protein components.

Prostaglandins – a group of fatty-acid derived lipid compounds that play an important role in inflammation.

Reverse transcriptase – enzyme important in viral replication.

Superoxide dismutase – one of a group of enzymes that are an important part of antioxidant defence in cells.

Th2 – T-helper Cell 2 – Immune cells involved in immune regulation and often described as promoting a pro-inflammatory immune response.

Triterpenes – compounds in the terpenoid class of organic molecules, which also contains essential oils.

References

1. Medicinal mushrooms: their therapeutic properties and current medical usage with special emphasis on cancer treatments. Smith J, Rowan N, Sullican R. May 2002 Report for Cancer Research UK.

2. Cancer Risk Reduction by Intake of Mushrooms and Clinical Studies on EEM. Ikekawa T. Int J Med Mush. 2005;7(3):347.

3. Medicinal mushroom science: history, current status, future trends and unsolved problems. Wasser SP. Int J Med Mushr. 2010;12(1):1-16.

4. A review on antimicrobial activity of mushroom (Basidiomycetes) extracts and isolated compounds. Alves MJ, Ferreira IC, Dias J, Teixeira V, Martins A, Pintado M. Planta Med. 2012 Nov;78(16):1707-18.

5. The effects of β-glucan on human immune and cancer cells. Chan GC, Chan WK and Sze MY. Journal of Hematology & Oncology 2009, 2:25.

6. Medicinal mushrooms as a source of antitumor and immunomodulating polysaccharides. Wasser SP. Appl. Environ Microbiol. 2002;60:258-274.

7. Antitumor activity of mushroom polysaccharides: a review. Ren L, Perera C, Hemar Y. Food Funct. 2012 Nov;3(11):1118-30.

8. Immunomodulatory dietary polysaccharides: a systematic review of the literature. Ramberg JE, Nelson ED, Sinnott RA. Nutr J. 2010 Nov 18;9:54.

9. Polysaccharide-rich fraction of *Agaricus brasiliensis* enhances the candidacidal activity of murine macrophages. Martins PR, Gameiro MC, Castoldi L, Romagnoli GG, Lopes FC, Pinto AV, Loyola W, Kaneno R. Mem Inst Oswaldo Cruz. 2008 May;103(3):244-50.

10. An examination of antibacterial and antifungal properties of constituents of Shiitake (*Lentinula edodes*) and oyster (*Pleurotus ostreatus*) mushrooms. Hearst R, Nelson D, McCollum G, Millar BC, Maeda Y, Goldsmith CE, Rooney PJ, Loughrey A, Rao JR, Moore JE. Complement Ther Clin Pract. 2009 Feb;15(1):5-7.

11. Protective effects of a protein-bound polysaccharide, PSK, on Candida albicans infection in mice via tumor necrosis factor-alpha induction. Ohmura Y, Matsunaga K, Motokawa I, Sakurai K, Ando T. Int Immunopharmacol. 2001 Sep;1(9-10):1797-811.

12. Dietary intakes of mushrooms and green tea combine to reduce the risk of breast cancer in Chinese women. Zhang M, Huang J, Xie X, Holman CD. Int J Cancer. 2009 Mar 15;124(6):1404-8.

13. Agaricus subrufescens: A review. Wisitrassameewong K *et al.* Saudi Journal of Biological Sciences. Volume 19, Issue 2, April 2012, Pages 131–146

14. Anti-aromatase activity of phytochemicals in white button mushrooms (*Agaricus bisporus*). Chen S *et al.* Cancer Res. 2006 Dec 15;66(24):12026-34.

15. Immunomodulating activity of *Agaricus brasiliensis* KA21 in mice and in human volunteers. Liu Y, Fukuwatari Y, Okumura K, Takeda K, Ishibashi KI, Furukawa M,

Ohno N, Mori K, Gao M, Motoi M. Evid Based Complement Alternat Med. 2008;5(2):205-219.

16. Natural killer cell activity and quality of life were improved by consumption of a mushroom extract, *Agaricus blazei* Murill Kyowa, in gynecological cancer patients undergoing chemotherapy. Ahn WS *et al*. Int J Gynecol Cancer 2004;14(4):589-594.

17. The medicinal mushroom *Agaricus blazei* Murrill: Review of literature and Pharmacotoxicological problems. Firenzuoli F, Gori L, Lombardo G. Evid Based Complement Alternat Med. 2008;5(1):3-15.

18. Medicinal properties and clinical effects of culinary-medicinal mushroom *Agaricus blazei* Murrill (Agaricomycetideae) (Review). Mizuno T. Int J Med Mushr 2002; 4:299–312.

19. The mushroom *Agaricus blazei* Murill extract normalizes liver function in patients with chronic hepatitis B. Hsu CH, Hwang KC, Chiang YH, Chou P. J Altern Complement Med. 2008;14(3):299-301.

20. The Chaga Storey. Spinosa R. 2006. The Mycophile, 47:1.

21. Plants used against cancer. Hartwell JL. 1982. Quartermain Pubs: Lawrence, Mass. p.694.

22. Chemistry, biological activity, and chemotherapeutic potential of betulinic acid for the prevention and treatment of cancer and HIV infection. Cichewicz RH, Kouzi SA. Med Res Rev. 2004;24(1):90-114.

23. Treatment of Psoriasis with Using Chaga Mushroom Preparations. Dosychev EA, Bystrova VN. 1973. Vestn Dermatol Venerol. May;47(5):79-83.

24. Medicinal value of the caterpillar fungi species of the genus Cordyceps (Fr.) Link (Ascomycetes). A Review. Holliday J, Cleaver M. Int J Med Mushr, 2008;10(3):219–234.

25. Effect of Cs-4® (*Cordyceps sinensis*) on Exercise Performance in Healthy Older Subjects: A Double-Blind, Placebo-Controlled Trial. Chen S, Li Z, Krochmal R, Abrazado M, Kim W, Cooper C. J Altern Complement Med. 2010 May; 16(5): 585–590.

26. Effect of medicinal plant extracts on forced swimming capacity in mice. Jung K, Kim IH, Han D. J Ethnopharmacol. 2004 Jul;93(1):75-81.

27. Hypoglycemic activity of polysaccharide, with antioxidation, isolated from cultured Cordyceps mycelia. Li SP, Zhang GH, Zeng Q, Huang ZG, Wang YT, Dong TT, Tsim KW. Phytomedicine. 2006 Jun;13(6):428-33.

28. Cordycepin Suppresses Expression of Diabetes Regulating Genes by Inhibition of Lipopolysaccharide-induced Inflammation in Macrophages. Shin S, Lee S, Kwon J, Moon S, Lee S, Lee CK, Cho K, Ha NJ, Kim K. Immune Netw. 2009 Jun;9(3):98-105.

29. Effect of long-term administration of cordycepin from *Cordyceps militaris* on testicular function in middle-aged rats. Sohn SH *et al*. Planta Med. 2012 Oct;78(15):1620-5.

30. Improvement of sperm production in subfertile boars by *Cordyceps militaris* supplement. Lin WH *et al*. Am J Chin Med. 2007;35(4):631-41.

31. Upregulation of Steroidogenic Enzymes and Ovarian 17β-Estradiol in Human Granulosa-Lutein Cells by *Cordyceps sinensis* Mycelium. Huang BM, Hsiao KY, Chuang PC, Wu MH, Pan HA, Tsai SJ. Biology of Reproduction May 1, 2004 vol. 70 no. 5 1358-1364.

32. Inhibitive Effect of *Cordyceps sinensis* on Experimental Hepatic Fibrosis and its Possible Mechanism – Liu YK, Shen W. World J Gastroenterol. 2003 Mar; 9(3):529-33.

33. The use of mushroom glucans and proteoglycans in cancer treatment. Parris K. Alternative Medicine Rev. 2000:5(1).

34. *Coriolus versicolor* – Detailed Scientific Review. MD Anderson Cancer Center.

35. Efficacy of Yun Zhi (*Coriolus versicolor*) on survival in cancer patients: systematic review and meta-analysis. Eliza WL, Fai CK, Chung LP. Recent Pat Inflamm Allergy Drug Discov. 2012 Jan;6(1):78-87.

36. Medicinal value of turkey tail fungus Trametes versicolor (L.:Fr.) Pilát (Aphyllophoro-mycetideae). A Literature Review. Christopher Hobbs. Int J Med Mushr 2004;6(3).

37. Coriolus. Munroe J. J Integrative Medicine. 2004;8:101-108.

38. The anti-dementia effect of Lion's Mane mushroom and its clinical application. Kawagishi H, Zhuang C, Shnidman E. Townsend Letter for Doctors and Patients, April 2004.

39. Improving effects of the mushroom Yamabushitake (*Hericium erinaceus*) on mild cognitive impairment: a double-blind placebo-controlled clinical trial. Mori K, Inatomi S, Ouchi K, Azumi Y, Tuchida T. Phytother Res. 2009;23(3):367-72.

40. Nerve growth factor and diabetic neuropathy. Pittenger G, Vinik A. Exp Diabesity Res. 2003;4(4):271-85. Review.

41. Long-term treatment with recombinant nerve growth factor for HIV-associated sensory neuropathy. Schifitto G *et al*. Neurology. 2001;57:1313-1316.

42. Neuroregenerative Potential of Lion's Mane Mushroom, *Hericium erinaceus* (Bull.: Fr.) Pers. (Higher Basidiomycetes), in the Treatment of Peripheral Nerve Injury (Review). Wong KH, Naidu M, David RP, Bakar R, Sabaratnam V. Int J Med Mushrooms, 2012; 14(5):427-446.

43. Erinacine E as a kappa opioid receptor agonist and its new analogs from a basidiomycete, *Hericium ramosum*. Saito T *et al*. J Antibiot (Tokyo). 1998 Nov; 51(11):983-90.

44. Anti-MRSA compounds of *Hericium erinaceus*. Kawagishi H *et al*. Int J Med Mushr. 2005;7(3):350.

45. *In vitro* anti-helicobacter pylori effects of medicinal mushroom extracts, with special emphasis on the Lion's Mane mushroom, *Hericium erinaceus* (higher Basidiomycetes). Shang X, Tan Q, Liu R, Yu K, Li P, Zhao GP. Int J Med Mushrooms. 2013;15(2):165-74.

46. Maitake extracts and their therapeutic potential – A review. Mayell M. Alt Med Rev, 2001;6(1).

47. *Grifola frondosa* (Dicks.: Fr.). Gray SF (Maitake Mushroom): medicinal properties,

active compounds, and biotechnological cultivation. Boh B, Berovic MM. Int J Med Mushr. 2007;9(2):10.

48. Maitake D-fraction: healing and preventive potential for cancer. Nanba H. J Orthomolecular Med. 1997;12:43-49.

49. Can Maitake MD-fraction aid cancer patients? Kodama N, Komuta K, Nanba H. Alt Med Rev. 2002;(7)3:236-9.

50. Chinese Medical Herbology and Pharmacology. Chen JK, Chen TT. 2001:386. Pub. Art of Medicine Press.

51. Anti-diabetic activity present in the fruit body of *Grifola frondosa* (Maitake). Kubo K, Aoki H, Nanba H. Biol Pharm Bull. 1994;17:1106-1110.

52. A possible hypoglycemic effect of maitake mushroom on type 2 diabetic patients. Konno S *et al*. Diabetic Med. 2001. Dec; 18(12):1010.

53. Polycystic ovary syndrome: a complex condition with psychological, reproductive and metabolic manifestations that impacts on health across the lifespan. Teede H, Deeks A and Moran L. BMC Medicine 2010, 8:41.

54. Maitake Mushroom (*Grifola frondosa*) Extract Induces Ovulation in Patients with Polycystic Ovary Syndrome: A Possible Monotherapy and a Combination Therapy After Failure with First-Line Clomiphene Citrate. Chen J *et al*. The Journal of Alternative and Complementary Medicine, Vol. 16, No. 12, 2010, pp. 1295-1299.

55. Lanostanes from *Phellinus igniarius* and their iNOS inhibitory activities. Wang GJ, Tsai TH, Chang TT, Chou CJ, Lin LC. Planta Med. 2009 Dec;75(15):1602-7.

56. Styrylpyrone-class compounds from medicinal fungi Phellinus and Inonotus spp., and their medicinal importance. Lee IK, Yun BS. J Antibiot (Tokyo). 2011 May;64(5):349-59.

57. Current advances in Phellinus sensu lato: medicinal species, functions, metabolites and mechanisms. Dai YC, Zhou LW, Cui BK, Chen YQ, Decock C. Appl Microbiol Biotechnol. 2010 Aug;87(5):1587-93.

58. A medicinal mushroom: *Phellinus linteus*. Zhu T, Kim SH, Chen CY. Curr Med Chem. 2008;15(13):1330-5.

59. Stimulation of humoral and cell mediated immunity by polysaccharides from mushroom Phellinus linteus. Kim HM *et al*. International Journal of Immunopharmacology, 1996 May; 18(5): 295-303.

60. Phellinus linteus extract augments the immune response in Mitomycin C-induced immunodeficient mice. Matsuba S, Matsuno H, Sakuma M, Komatsu Y. Evid Based Complement Alternat Med. 2008;5(1):85-90.6.

61. Effect of *Phellius linteus* water extract on benign prostatic hyperplasia. Kim YN, Kim MS, Chun SS, Choi JH. Nutr Res Pract. 2013 Jun;7(3):172-7.

62. Immune Related Female Infertility. Wing T. TCM Kongress Rothenburg 2012.

63. Oral administration of proteoglycan isolated from *Phellinus linteus* in the prevention and treatment of collagen-induced arthritis in mice. Kim GY *et al*. Biol Pharm Bull. 2003;26(6):823-31.

64. Antiarthritic activity of a Polysaccharide-protein complex isolated from *Phellinus rimosus* (Berk.) Pilát (Aphyllophoromycetideae) in Freund's complete adjuvant-induced arthritic rats. Meera CR, Smina TP, Nitha B, Mathew J, Janardhanan KK. Int J Med Mushr. 2009;11(1):21-28.

65. Inhibition of anaphylaxis-like reaction and mast cell activation by water extract from the fruiting body of *Phellinus linteus*. Choi YH, Yan GH, Chai OH, Lim JM, Sung SY, Zhang X, Kim JH, Choi SH, Lee MS, Han EH, Kim HT, Song CH. Biol Pharm Bull. 2006 Jul;29(7):1360-5.

66. Ganoderma – a therapeutic fungal biofactory. Paterson RR. Phytochemistry. 2006; 67(18):1985-2001.

67. Anticancer effects of *Ganoderma lucidum*: a review of scientific evidence. Yuen JW, Gohel MD. Nutr Cancer. 2005;53(1):11-7.

68. *Ganoderma lucidum* (Reishi mushroom) for cancer treatment. Jin X, Ruiz Beguerie J, Sze DM, Chan GC. Cochrane Database Syst Rev. 2012 Jun 13;6:CD007731.

69. *Ganoderma lucidum* and its pharmaceutically active compounds. Boh B, Berovic M, Zhang J, Zhi-Bin L. Biotechnol Annu Rev. 2007;13:265-301.

70. The use of *Ganoderma lucidum* (Reishi) in the management of Histamine-mediated allergic responses. Powell M. The Nutrition Practitioner. October 2004.

71. A preliminary study on the sleep-improvement function of the effective ingredients of *Ganoderma lucidum* fruitbody. Jia W, Wu M, Zhang JS, Liu YF. Acta Edulis Fungi. 2005;12(3):43-47.

72. A phase I/II study of ling zhi mushroom *Ganoderma lucidum* (W.Curt.:Fr.) Lloyd (Aphyllophoromycetideae) extract in patients with coronary heart disease. Gao Y, Chen G, Dai X, Ye J, Zhou S. Int J Med Mushrooms 2004;6(4):30.

73. Medicinal Mushrooms – An Exploration of Tradition, Healing and Culture. Hobbs C. 1986. Pub. Botanica Press, Williams. p.96-107.

74. Efficacy of S-adenosylhomocysteine hydrolase inhibitors, D-eritadenine and (S)-DHPA, against the growth of Cryptosporidium parvum *in vitro*. Vlasta Čtrnáctá,1,2 Fritzler JM, Šurinová M, Hrdý I, Zhu G, and Stejskal F. Exp Parasitol. 2010 October; 126(2): 113–116.

75. Shiitake (*Lentinus edodes*) Wasser SP. Encyclopedia of Dietary Supplements 2nd Ed. 2010. Pub. Informa Healthcare. p.719-726.

76. Individual patient based meta-analysis of lentinan for unresectable/recurrent gastric cancer. Oba K, Kobayashi M, Matsui T, Kodera Y, Sakamoto J. Anticancer Res. 2009;29(7):2739-45.

77. The medicinal benefits of Lentinan (β-1, 3-D glucan) from *Lentinus edodes* (Berk.) singer (Shiitake Mushroom) through oral administration. Yap AT, Ng MH. Int J Med Mushr. 2005;7(12):170.

78. Medicinal value of the genus Tremella Pers. (Heterobasidiomycetes) (Review). Reshetnikov SV, Wasser SP, Duckman I, and Tsukor K. 2000. Int J Med Mushr. 2000;2:345-367.

79. Research advances in primary biological effects of Tremella polysaccharides. Chen FF, Cai DL. Zhong Xi Yi Jie He Xue Bao. 2008;6(8):862-6.

80. Effect of polysaccharides from *Auricularia auricula* underw, *Tremella fuciformis* Berk and spores of *Tremella fuciformis* Berk on ageing. Chen YJ *et al*. Chinese Journal of Modern Applied Pharmacy. 1989-02.

81. *Ganoderma lucidum* inhibits proliferation and induces apoptosis in human prostate cancer cells PC-3. Jiang J, Slivova V, Valachovicova T, Harvey K and Sliva D. Int J Oncol 2004; 24: 1093-1099.

82. The cancer preventive effects of edible mushrooms. Xu T, Beelman RB, Lambert JD. Anticancer Agents Med Chem. 2012 Dec;12(10):1255-63.

83. A case-control study on the dietary intake of mushrooms and breast cancer risk among Korean women. Hong SA, Kim K, Nam SJ, Kong G, Kim MK. Int J Cancer. 2008 Feb 15;122(4):919-23.

84. *Coriolus versicolor* supplementation in HPV patients, Couto S, Da Silva DP. 20th European Congress of Obstetrics and Gynaecology. 2008.

85. Efficacy of adjuvant immunochemotherapy with polysaccharide K for patients with curatively resected colorectal cancer: a meta-analysis of centrally randomized controlled clinical trials. Sakamoto J *et al*. Cancer Immunol Immunother. 2006 Apr;55(4):404-11.

86. Monitoring of immune responses to a herbal immuno-modulator in patients with advanced colorectal cancer. Chen X *et al*. Int Immunopharmacol. 2006 Mar;6(3): 499-508.

87. *Coriolus versicolor* polysaccharide peptide slows progression of advanced non-small cell lung cancer. Tsang KW et al. Respir Med. 2003 Jun;97(6):618-24.

88. RNA-directed agent, cordycepin, induces cell death in multiple myeloma cells. Chen LS, Stellrecht CM, Gandhi V. Br J Haematol. 2008 Mar;140(6):682-391.

89. Personal communication. Prof. Yumin He – Director of Chinese Medical Association, Shanghai University of TCM.

90. Pharmacological values of medicinal mushrooms for prostate cancer therapy: the case of *Ganoderma lucidum*. Mahajna J, Dotan N, Zaidman BZ, Petrova RD, Wasser SP. Nutr Cancer. 2009;61(1):16-26.

91. Immunomodulatory effect of pleuran (β-glucan from *Pleurotus ostreatus*) in children with recurrent respiratory tract infections. Jesenak M et al. Int Immunopharmacol. 2013 Feb;15(2):395-9.

92. Comparative study of contents of several bioactive components in fruiting bodies and mycelia of culinary-medicinal mushrooms. Lin SY *et al*. Int J Med Mushrooms. 2013;15(3):315-23.

93. *Cordyceps sinensis* supplementation in alcohol-induced liver steatosis. Santos C. Mycology News, 2004;1(9).

94. Evaluation of the hepatic and renal-protective effects of *Ganoderma lucidum* in mice. Shieh H *et al*. Am J Chin Med. 2001;29(3-4):501-7.

Index

Further Reading

Reishi Mushroom – Herb of Spiritual Potency and Medical Wonder. Willard T. Sylvan Press 1990. *Out of print*

Medicinal Mushrooms – An Exploration of Tradition, Healing and Culture. Hobbs C. Botanica Press 1995.

Growing Gourmet and Medicinal Mushrooms, 3rd Ed. Stamets P. Ten Speed Press 2000.

Medicinal Mushrooms – Ancient Remedies for Modern Ailments. Halpern G. M. Evans & Company 2002. *Out of print*

Mycelium Running – How Mushrooms can save the World. Stamets P. One Speed Press 2004.

Healing Mushrooms – Effective Treatments for Today's Illnesses. Halpern G. One Speed Press 2007.

Medicinal Mushrooms – A Clinical Guide. Powell M. Mycology Press 2010.

The Fungal Pharmacy – The Complete Guide to the Medicinal Mushrooms and Lichens of North America. Rogers R. North Atlantic Books 2011.

Chaga – The King of Medicinal Mushrooms. Wolfe D. North Atlantic Books 2012.